JUICING TO BOOST FERTILITY

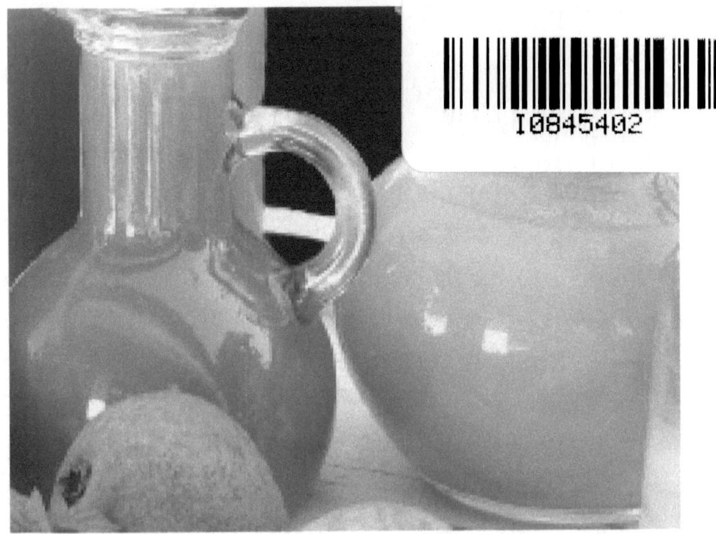

20 Nutritious Fruit Extracts to Boost the Immune System and Enhance Reproduction

Lincoln Kimmons

Juicing to Boost Fertility

Table of Content

Introduction

Have you ever experienced a deep need that appears to exist beyond time, the echo of longing? That was an all too familiar sensation. I found myself searching for a new type of nourishment—one that went beyond simple nutrition and offered the promise of life—in a world where the pleasure of motherhood remained unattainable.

I danced under the shadow of infertility, my heart heavy with uncountable letdowns. Parenthood's hushed promises seemed like they were slipping through my fingers. At this emotional moment, I came onto a plethora of juicing recipes, many of which whispered stories of fertility and fresh starts.

Curious, I set out on a voyage through colorful mixtures, each drink a communion with optimism. The rainbow of fruits and vegetables turned into my allies; they were a symphony of tastes that matched the pulse of life. I experienced a subtle change as I included

these elixirs into my daily routine—a renewal
that went beyond the physical.

Day by day, I felt a blossoming within, a coming
back of optimism, a calm confidence that
defied the confines of medical prognosis. The
juice recipes were no longer just remedies;
they were forces for change. My body
synchronized with the nutrient-dense elixirs,
reflecting my regenerated energy.

A few months later, the sound of a beating
heart became my bedtime story, and the nest
of my dreams contained the priceless
happiness I had long yearned for. The juice
recipes, which had previously been a collection
of ingredients, had now written a new chapter
in my story. I had weaved a story of
overcoming hardship in the vast fabric of life,
which is evidence of the transformational force
found in the embrace of nature.

In addition to my kid, I became a mother to the
unbreakable optimism that lives in every
optimistic heart. I turned to face the light that
had been sparked within me, just as
sunflowers unfolded toward the sun. This
beautiful glow was nourished by seeds of

optimism and hydrated by the soft cascade of a juiced symphony."

Chapter 1

Nutritious Recipes

Berry Boost

Ingredients:

- 1 cup strawberries, hulled
- 1/2 cup blueberries
- 1/2 cup raspberries
- 1/2 cup blackberries
- 1 medium-sized apple, cored and sliced
- 1 tablespoon chia seeds
- 1-2 teaspoons honey (optional, depending on sweetness preference)
- 1 cup cold water or coconut water
- Ice cubes (optional)

Instructions:

- Wash all the berries thoroughly.
- In a blender, combine strawberries, blueberries, raspberries, blackberries, apple slices, chia seeds, and cold water or coconut water.

- Blend until smooth and well combined. You may adjust the consistency by adding more water if it's too thick.
- Taste the mixture and add honey if additional sweetness is desired. Blend again to incorporate.
- Optional: Add ice cubes and blend once more for a refreshing chill.
- Pour the Berry Boost juice into the glasses.
- Garnish with a few whole berries on top for a visually appealing touch.

Nutritional Information (per serving):

- Calories: Approximately 150
- Fiber: 10g
- Vitamin C: 120% DV
- Antioxidants: High

Preparation Time: 10 minutes

Serving Suggestion:

- Enjoy in the morning for a nutrient-packed start.

Green Goddess

Ingredients:

- 2 cups kale, stems removed
- 1 cucumber, peeled and sliced
- 2 green apples, cored and sliced
- 1/2 lemon, peeled
- 1-inch piece of ginger, peeled
- 1 celery stalk
- 1 cup spinach leaves
- 1 cup cold coconut water or water
- Ice cubes (optional)

Instructions:

- Wash all vegetables and fruits thoroughly.
- In a blender, combine kale, cucumber, green apples, lemon, ginger, celery, spinach, and cold coconut water or water.
- Blend until smooth and well combined. If necessary, adjust the consistency by adding more water.
- Optional: Add ice cubes and blend again for a refreshing chill.
- Pour the Green Goddess juice into glasses.

Juicing to Boost Fertility

Nutritional Information (per serving):

- Calories: Approximately 120
- Vitamin A: 200% DV
- Vitamin C: 150% DV
- Iron: 15% DV

Preparation Time: 12 minutes

Serving Suggestion:

- Ideal for an afternoon energy boost.

Citrus Delight

Ingredients:

- 2 oranges, peeled and segmented
- 2 grapefruits, peeled and segmented
- 3 lemons, peeled
- 1 lime, peeled
- 1 tablespoon honey or agave syrup (optional, depending on sweetness preference)
- 1 cup cold water or coconut water
- Ice cubes (optional)

Instructions:

- Peel and segment the oranges and grapefruits.
- In a blender, combine the orange segments, grapefruit segments, peeled lemons, peeled lime, honey or agave syrup, and cold water or coconut water.
- Blend until smooth and well combined. Adjust sweetness by adding more honey or agave if desired.
- Optional: Add ice cubes and blend again for a cool, refreshing touch.
- Pour the Citrus Delight juice into glasses.

Nutritional Information (per serving):

- Calories: Approximately 100
- Vitamin C: 250% DV
- Potassium: 10% DV
- Folate: 15% DV

Preparation Time: 15 minutes

Serving Suggestion:

- A refreshing drink for midday hydration.

Pomegranate Passion

Ingredients:

- 2 cups fresh pomegranate seeds
- 1 cup pineapple chunks
- 1 orange, peeled and segmented
- 1 tablespoon fresh mint leaves
- 1 tablespoon honey or agave syrup (optional, depending on sweetness preference)
- 1 cup cold water or coconut water
- Ice cubes (optional)

Instructions:

- Extract fresh pomegranate seeds and set aside.
- In a blender, combine pomegranate seeds, pineapple chunks, orange segments, fresh mint leaves, honey or agave syrup, and cold water or coconut water.
- Blend until smooth and well combined. Adjust sweetness by adding more honey or agave if desired.
- Optional: Add ice cubes and blend again for a chilled, refreshing texture.

- Pour the Pomegranate Passion juice into glasses.

Nutritional Information (per serving):

- Calories: Approximately 140
- Vitamin C: 100% DV
- Fiber: 5g
- Antioxidants: High

Preparation Time: 15 minutes

Serving Suggestion:

- Drink post-workout for recovery.

Carrot Zing

Ingredients:

- 4 large carrots, peeled and sliced
- 1 apple, cored and sliced
- 1-inch piece of ginger, peeled
- 1 lemon, peeled
- 1 tablespoon turmeric powder (optional for an extra zing)
- 1 tablespoon honey or agave syrup (optional, depending on sweetness preference)

- 1 cup cold water or coconut water
- Ice cubes (optional)

Instructions:

- Peel and slice the carrots, core and slice the apple, peel the ginger and lemon.
- In a blender, combine carrots, apple slices, ginger, lemon, turmeric powder (if using), honey or agave syrup, and cold water or coconut water.
- Blend until smooth and well combined. Adjust sweetness by adding more honey or agave if desired.
- Optional: Add ice cubes and blend again for a refreshing chill.
- Pour the Carrot Zing juice into glasses.

Nutritional Information (per serving):

- Calories: Approximately 120
- Vitamin A: 400% DV
- Vitamin C: 80% DV
- Potassium: 10% DV

Preparation Time: 12 minutes

Serving Suggestion:

Juicing to Boost Fertility

- Great as a morning pick-me-up.

Spinach Vitality

Ingredients:

- 2 cups fresh spinach leaves
- 1 cucumber, peeled and sliced
- 2 green apples, cored and sliced
- 1/2 lemon, peeled
- 1-inch piece of ginger, peeled
- 1 tablespoon chia seeds
- 1 tablespoon honey or agave syrup (optional, depending on sweetness preference)
- 1 cup cold water or coconut water
- Ice cubes (optional)

Instructions:

- Wash spinach leaves thoroughly.
- In a blender, combine spinach leaves, cucumber, green apples, lemon, ginger, chia seeds, honey or agave syrup, and cold water or coconut water.
- Blend until smooth and well combined. Adjust sweetness by adding more honey or agave if desired.

Juicing to Boost Fertility

- Optional: Add ice cubes and blend again for a refreshing chill.
- Pour the Spinach Vitality juice into glasses.

Nutritional Information (per serving):

- Calories: Approximately 130
- Vitamin A: 150% DV
- Vitamin C: 80% DV
- Iron: 15% DV

Preparation Time: 10 minutes

Serving Suggestion:

- Perfect for a pre-dinner boost.

Gingered Greens

Ingredients:

- 3 cups kale, stems removed
- 1 cucumber, peeled and sliced
- 2 green apples, cored and sliced
- 1-inch piece of ginger, peeled
- 1/2 lemon, peeled
- 1 tablespoon chia seeds

- 1 tablespoon honey or agave syrup (optional, depending on sweetness preference)
- 1 cup cold water or coconut water
- Ice cubes (optional)

Instructions:

- Wash kale leaves thoroughly and remove stems.
- In a blender, combine kale, cucumber, green apples, ginger, lemon, chia seeds, honey or agave syrup, and cold water or coconut water.
- Blend until smooth and well combined. Adjust sweetness by adding more honey or agave if desired.
- Optional: Add ice cubes and blend again for a refreshing chill.
- Pour the GinGingereen juice into glasses.

Nutritional Information (per serving):

- Calories: Approximately 140
- Vitamin A: 200% DV
- Vitamin C: 100% DV
- Iron: 10% DV

Preparation Time: 12 minutes

Serving Suggestion:

- Enjoy in the afternoon for a digestive aid.

Fertility Fusion

Ingredients:

- 1 cup pineapple chunks
- 1 cup mango chunks
- 1 banana
- 1/2 avocado
- 1 tablespoon flaxseeds
- 1 tablespoon honey or agave syrup (optional, depending on sweetness preference)
- 1 cup almond milk or coconut water
- Ice cubes (optional)

Instructions:

- Peel and chop pineapple, mango, and banana.
- Scoop out the avocado.
- In a blender, combine pineapple chunks, mango chunks, banana, avocado,

flaxseeds, honey or agave syrup, and
almond milk or coconut water.

- Blend until smooth and well combined.
  Adjust sweetness by adding more honey
  or agave if desired.
- Optional: Add ice cubes and blend again
  for a refreshing chill.
- Pour the Fertility Fusion juice into
  glasses.

Nutritional Information (per serving):

- Calories: Approximately 250
- Vitamin C: 80% DV
- Folate: 30% DV
- Healthy Fats: High

Preparation Time: 10 minutes

Serving Suggestion:

- A tropical treat for any time of the day.

Cucumber Bliss

Ingredients:

- 2 cucumbers, peeled and sliced
- 1 green apple, cored and sliced

- 1/2 lime, peeled
- 1 cup fresh mint leaves
- 1 tablespoon chia seeds
- 1 tablespoon honey or agave syrup (optional, depending on sweetness preference)
- 1 cup cold water or coconut water
- Ice cubes (optional)

Instructions:

- Peel and slice the cucumbers.
- Core and slice the green apple.
- Peel the lime.
- In a blender, combine cucumber slices, green apple slices, peeled lime, fresh mint leaves, chia seeds, honey or agave syrup, and cold water or coconut water.
- Blend until smooth and well combined. Adjust sweetness by adding more honey or agave if desired.
- Optional: Add ice cubes and blend again for a refreshing chill.
- Pour the Cucumber Bliss juice into glasses.

Nutritional Information (per serving):

- Calories: Approximately 100

Juicing to Boost Fertility

- Vitamin A: 10% DV
- Vitamin C: 50% DV
- Hydration: High

Preparation Time: 8 minutes

Serving Suggestion:
- A refreshing drink for hot afternoons.

Beet Berry Boost

Ingredients:

- 1 medium-sized beetroot, peeled and chopped
- 1 cup mixed berries (strawberries, blueberries, raspberries, blackberries)
- 1 apple, cored and sliced
- 1/2 lemon, peeled
- 1 tablespoon chia seeds
- 1 tablespoon honey or agave syrup (optional, depending on sweetness preference)
- 1 cup cold water or coconut water
- Ice cubes (optional)

Instructions:

- Peel and chop the beetroot.

Juicing to Boost Fertility

- In a blender, combine chopped beetroot, mixed berries, apple slices, peeled lemon, chia seeds, honey or agave syrup, and cold water or coconut water.
- Blend until smooth and well combined. Adjust sweetness by adding more honey or agave if desired.
- Optional: Add ice cubes and blend again for a refreshing chill.
- Pour the Beet Berry Boost juice into glasses.

Nutritional Information (per serving):

- Calories: Approximately 120
- Fiber: 8g
- Vitamin C: 90% DV
- Iron: 10% DV

Preparation Time: 15 minutes

Serving Suggestion:

- Perfect as a digestive help after a meal.

Turmeric Tonic

Ingredients:

- 2 large carrots, peeled and sliced
- 1 orange, peeled and segmented
- 1-inch piece of turmeric, peeled
- 1/2 lemon, peeled
- 1 tablespoon fresh ginger, peeled and grated
- 1 tablespoon honey or agave syrup (optional, depending on sweetness preference)
- 1 cup cold water or coconut water
- Ice cubes (optional)

Instructions:

- Peel and slice the carrots, peel the orange and lemon, and grate the ginger.
- In a blender, combine carrot slices, orange segments, peeled turmeric, peeled lemon, grated ginger, honey or agave syrup, and cold water or coconut water.
- Blend until smooth and well combined. Adjust sweetness by adding more honey or agave if desired.
- Optional: Add ice cubes and blend again for a refreshing chill.
- Pour the Turmeric Tonic juice into glasses.

Juicing to Boost Fertility

Nutritional Information (per serving):

- Calories: Approximately 110
- Vitamin C: 80% DV
- Anti-Inflammatory Properties: High

Preparation Time: 12 minutes

Serving Suggestion:

- Enjoy it with breakfast for an ideal beginning.

Folate Fizz

Ingredients:

- 1 cup kale, stems removed
- 1 cup spinach leaves
- 1 orange, peeled and segmented
- 1 banana
- 1/2 avocado
- 1 tablespoon flaxseeds
- 1 tablespoon honey or agave syrup (optional, depending on sweetness preference)
- 1 cup cold water or coconut water
- Sparkling water (to add fizz)
- Ice cubes (optional)

Juicing to Boost Fertility

Instructions:

- Wash kale and spinach leaves thoroughly.
- Peel and segment the orange.
- In a blender, combine kale, spinach leaves, orange segments, banana, avocado, flaxseeds, honey or agave syrup, and cold water or coconut water.
- Blend until smooth and well combined.
- Pour the juice into glasses, leaving some space at the top.
- Top up with sparkling water to add fizz.
- Optional: Add ice cubes for a refreshing chill.

Nutritional Information (per serving):

- Calories: Approximately 180
- Folate: 40% DV
- Vitamin C: 100% DV

Preparation Time: 10 minutes

Serving Suggestion:

- A cool option for a midday boost

Papaya Power

Ingredients:

- 2 cups ripe papaya, peeled, seeded, and cubed
- 1 cup pineapple chunks
- 1 orange, peeled and segmented
- 1/2 lime, peeled
- 1 tablespoon fresh mint leaves
- 1 tablespoon honey or agave syrup (optional, depending on sweetness preference)
- 1 cup cold coconut water or water
- Ice cubes (optional)

Instructions:

- Peel, seed, and cube the ripe papaya.
- In a blender, combine papaya cubes, pineapple chunks, orange segments, peeled lime, fresh mint leaves, honey or agave syrup, and cold coconut water or water.
- Blend until smooth and well combined. Adjust sweetness by adding more honey or agave if desired.
- Optional: Add ice cubes and blend again for a refreshing chill.

Juicing to Boost Fertility

- Pour the Papaya Power juice into glasses.

Nutritional Information (per serving):

- Calories: Approximately 120
- Vitamin C: 150% DV
- Vitamin A: 60% DV

Preparation Time: 12 minutes

Serving Suggestion:

- Perfect as a post-exercise refreshment.

Orange Blossom

Ingredients:

- 4 oranges, peeled and segmented
- 1 grapefruit, peeled and segmented
- 1 lemon, peeled
- 1 tablespoon honey or agave syrup (optional, depending on sweetness preference)
- 1 tablespoon fresh mint leaves
- 1 cup cold water or coconut water
- Ice cubes (optional)

Instructions:

- Peel and cut the lemon, grapefruit, and oranges into segments.
- In a blender, combine orange segments, grapefruit segments, peeled lemon, honey or agave syrup, fresh mint leaves, and cold water or coconut water.
- Blend until smooth and well combined. Adjust sweetness by adding more honey or agave if desired.
- Optional: Add ice cubes and blend again for a refreshing chill.
- Pour the Orange Blossom juice into glasses.

Nutritional Information (per serving):

- Calories: Approximately 110
- Vitamin C: 150% DV
- Antioxidants: High

Preparation Time: 10 minutes

Serving Suggestion:

- Great as a morning energy boost.

Blueberry Bliss

Ingredients:

- 1 cup blueberries
- 1 cup strawberries, hulled
- 1 banana
- 1/2 cup Greek yogurt (optional for creaminess)
- 1 tablespoon honey or agave syrup (optional, depending on sweetness preference)
- 1 cup cold almond milk or coconut water
- Ice cubes (optional)

Instructions:

- Wash blueberries and strawberries thoroughly.
- In a blender, combine blueberries, strawberries, banana, Greek yogurt (if using), honey or agave syrup, and cold almond milk or coconut water.
- Blend until smooth and well combined. Adjust sweetness by adding more honey or agave if desired.
- Optional: Add ice cubes and blend again for a refreshing chill.

Juicing to Boost Fertility

- Pour the Blueberry Bliss juice into the glasses.

Nutritional Information (per serving):

- Calories: Approximately 180
- Fiber: 5g
- Vitamin C: 80% DV
- Antioxidants: High

Preparation Time: 8 minutes

Serving Suggestion:

- Ideal for a cool-down after yoga.

Mango Melody

Ingredients:

- 2 ripe mangoes, peeled and diced
- 1 cup pineapple chunks
- 1 banana
- 1/2 lime, peeled
- 1 tablespoon chia seeds
- 1 tablespoon honey or agave syrup (optional, depending on sweetness preference)
- 1 cup cold coconut water or water

- Ice cubes (optional)

Instructions:
- Peel and dice the ripe mangoes.
- In a blender, combine diced mangoes, pineapple chunks, banana, peeled lime, chia seeds, honey or agave syrup, and cold coconut water or water.
- Blend until smooth and well combined. Adjust sweetness by adding more honey or agave if desired.
- Optional: Add ice cubes and blend again for a refreshing chill.
- Pour the Mango Melody juice into glasses.

Nutritional Information (per serving):

- Calories: Approximately 160
- Vitamin C: 90% DV
- Fiber: 7g

Preparation Time: 10 minutes

Serving Suggestion:

- A delicious afternoon treat.

Cherry Charm

Ingredients:

- 2 cups fresh cherries, pitted
- 1 cup red grapes
- 1 apple, cored and sliced
- 1/2 lemon, peeled
- 1 tablespoon honey or agave syrup (optional, depending on sweetness preference)
- 1 cup cold water or coconut water
- Ice cubes (optional)

Instructions:

- Pit the fresh cherries.
- In a blender, combine pitted cherries, red grapes, apple slices, peeled lemon, honey or agave syrup, and cold water or coconut water.
- Blend until smooth and well combined. Adjust sweetness by adding more honey or agave if desired.
- Optional: Add ice cubes and blend again for a refreshing chill.
- Pour the Cherry Charm juice into glasses.

Juicing to Boost Fertility

Nutritional Information (per serving):

- Calories: Approximately 120
- Vitamin C: 50% DV
- Antioxidants: High

Preparation Time: 12 minutes

Serving Suggestion:

- A delightful treat for any time of day.

Pineapple Pleasure

Ingredients:

- 2 cups fresh pineapple chunks
- 1 orange, peeled and segmented
- 1 banana
- 1/2 lime, peeled
- 1 tablespoon fresh mint leaves
- 1 tablespoon honey or agave syrup (optional, depending on sweetness preference)
- 1 cup cold coconut water or water
- Ice cubes (optional)

Instructions:

- Peel and cut the fresh pineapple into chunks.
- In a blender, combine pineapple chunks, orange segments, banana, peeled lime, fresh mint leaves, honey or agave syrup, and cold coconut water or water.
- Blend until smooth and well combined. Adjust sweetness by adding more honey or agave if desired.
- Optional: Add ice cubes and blend again for a refreshing chill.
- Pour the Pineapple Pleasure juice into glasses.

Nutritional Information (per serving):

- Calories: Approximately 150
- Vitamin C: 120% DV
- Manganese: 10% DV

Preparation Time: 10 minutes

Serving Suggestion:

- A cool option for warm days

Grapefruit Greenery

Ingredients:

- 2 grapefruits, peeled and segmented
- 2 cups kale, stems removed
- 1 cucumber, peeled and sliced
- 1 green apple, cored and sliced
- 1 tablespoon fresh mint leaves
- 1 tablespoon honey or agave syrup (optional, depending on sweetness preference)
- 1 cup cold water or coconut water
- Ice cubes (optional)

Instructions:

- Peel and segment the grapefruits.
- Wash kale leaves thoroughly and remove stems.
- In a blender, combine grapefruit segments, kale, cucumber, green apple slices, fresh mint leaves, honey or agave syrup, and cold water or coconut water.
- Blend until smooth and well combined. Adjust sweetness by adding more honey or agave if desired.
- Optional: Add ice cubes and blend again for a refreshing chill.
- Pour the Grapefruit Greenery juice into glasses.

Nutritional Information (per serving):

- Calories: Approximately 130
- Vitamin A: 150% DV
- Vitamin C: 120% DV
- Iron: 10% DV

Preparation Time: 12 minutes

Serving Suggestion:

- Perfect for rehydrating after exercise.

Cranberry Crush

Ingredients:

- 1 cup fresh or frozen cranberries
- 1 orange, peeled and segmented
- 1 apple, cored and sliced
- 1/2 lemon, peeled
- 1 tablespoon chia seeds
- 1 tablespoon honey or agave syrup (optional, depending on sweetness preference)
- 1 cup cold water or coconut water
- Ice cubes (optional)

Instructions:

- In a blender, combine cranberries, orange segments, apple slices, peeled lemon, chia seeds, honey or agave syrup, and cold water or coconut water.
- Blend until smooth and well combined. Adjust sweetness by adding more honey or agave if desired.
- Optional: Add ice cubes and blend again for a refreshing chill.
- Pour the Cranberry Crush juice into glasses.

Nutritional Information (per serving):

- Calories: Approximately 120
- Vitamin C: 80% DV
- Antioxidants: High

Preparation Time: 10 minutes

Serving Suggestion:

- Excellent as a morning kickstart

Conclusion

In conclusion, the carefully chosen recipe book consisting of recipes that increase fertility, is meant to provide an approach to reproductive health. Readers may actively support their reproductive systems by adding nutrient-dense fruits, vegetables, and superfoods into these drinks.

Readers who set out on this path to better fertility are embracing a lifestyle that emphasizes nutrition for the health of their reproductive system rather than merely changing their food. These recipes are not just a list of drinks; they are a guide to a diet that supports fertility. Adherence to these recipes with consistency may help improve general health and fertility.

This book is a useful resource for anybody aspiring to become a parent since it provides not only scrumptious and revitalizing recipes but also a feeling of control over one's reproductive health. The satisfaction of providing the body with healthful foods and the possibility of favorable results inspire readers to embrace these recipes and make them part

Juicing to Boost Fertility

of their everyday routines. May those pursuing parenting find this journey to be a life-changing experience that gives them energy and hope.

We appreciate you looking at "Juicing to Boost Fertility." We appreciate your dedication to unlocking these recipes' potential. May you find pleasure and vigor on your path to improved fertility. Cheers to your health and the opportunities that lay ahead.

Bonus

1. Butterfly Pose (Baddha Konasana): Sit with your feet together, allowing your knees to sag slightly to the floor to increase hip and groin flexibility.

2. Child's Pose (Balasana): Kneel on the mat, sit back on your heels, and extend your arms forward so that your forehead rests on the ground. This position extends the lower back and encourages relaxation.

3. Pelvic Tilts: To contract and relax the pelvic muscles, lie on your back with your legs bent. Gently tilt your pelvis up and down.

4. The seated forward bend (paschimottanasana): strengthens the hamstrings and spine by having you sit with your legs out in front of you, hinge at the hips, and reach for your toes.

5. Cat-Cow Stretch: To increase spine flexibility and mobility, alternately round and arch your back while on your hands and knees.

Juicing to Boost Fertility

6. Legs Up the Wall Pose (Viparita Karani):
This pose eases tension, improves circulation, and promotes relaxation. It is performed on your back against a wall.

7. Reclining Bound Angle Pose (Supta Baddha Konasana): With your knees bent to the sides and your feet together, it encourages well-being and relaxation.

8. Low Lunge (Anjaneyasana): To increase hip flexibility and stretch the groin, step forward into a lunge stance with one foot.

9. Mountain Pose (Tadasana): To develop balance and strength, stand erect with your feet together, ground yourself, and concentrate on your breathing.

10. Meditation: To lower stress and improve general well-being, choose a comfortable seat, pay attention to your breathing, and practice mindfulness meditation.

Happy Juicing!!